T0320718

Cambridge Elements ≡

Elements in Emergency Neurosurgery
edited by
Nihal Gurusinghe
Lancashire Teaching Hospital NHS Trust
Peter Hutchinson
University of Cambridge, Society of British Neurological Surgeons and Royal College of Surgeons of England
Ioannis Fouyas
Royal College of Surgeons of Edinburgh
Naomi Slator
North Bristol NHS Trust
Ian Kamaly-Asl
Royal Manchester Children's Hospital
Peter Whitfield
University Hospitals Plymouth NHS Trust

CLINICAL PRIORITY FOR COMMON EMERGENCY AND URGENT CONDITIONS IN NEUROSURGERY

Taha Lilo
Royal Preston Hospital
Ioannis Fouyas
Royal College of Surgeons of Edinburgh

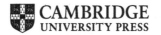

CAMBRIDGE
UNIVERSITY PRESS

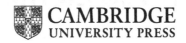

Shaftesbury Road, Cambridge CB2 8EA, United Kingdom

One Liberty Plaza, 20th Floor, New York, NY 10006, USA

477 Williamstown Road, Port Melbourne, VIC 3207, Australia

314–321, 3rd Floor, Plot 3, Splendor Forum, Jasola District Centre, New Delhi – 110025, India

103 Penang Road, #05–06/07, Visioncrest Commercial, Singapore 238467

Cambridge University Press is part of Cambridge University Press & Assessment, a department of the University of Cambridge.

We share the University's mission to contribute to society through the pursuit of education, learning and research at the highest international levels of excellence.

www.cambridge.org
Information on this title: www.cambridge.org/9781009486026

DOI: 10.1017/9781009440615

First published 2024

A catalogue record for this publication is available from the British Library.

ISBN 978-1-009-48602-6 Hardback
ISBN 978-1-009-44063-9 Paperback
ISSN 2755-0656 (online)
ISSN 2755-0648 (print)

Cambridge University Press & Assessment has no responsibility for the persistence or accuracy of URLs for external or third-party internet websites referred to in this publication and does not guarantee that any content on such websites is, or will remain, accurate or appropriate.

Every effort has been made in preparing this Element to provide accurate and up-to-date information which is in accord with accepted standards and practice at the time of publication. Although case histories are drawn from actual cases, every effort has been made to disguise the identities of the individuals involved. Nevertheless, the authors, editors and publishers can make no warranties that the information contained herein is totally free from error, not least because clinical standards are constantly changing through research and regulation. The authors, editors and publishers therefore disclaim all liability for direct or consequential damages resulting from the use of material contained in this Element. Readers are strongly advised to pay careful attention to information provided by the manufacturer of any drugs or equipment that they plan to use.

Clinical Priority for Common Emergency and Urgent Conditions in Neurosurgery

Elements in Emergency Neurosurgery

DOI: 10.1017/9781009440615
First published online: April 2024

Taha Lilo
Royal Preston Hospital

Ioannis Fouyas
Royal College of Surgeons of Edinburgh

Author for correspondence: Ioannis Fouyas, ifouyas@yahoo.com

Abstract: Emergency Neurosurgery is a constantly evolving specialty, resulting in ever-increasing challenges posed on the higher specialty trainee. The focus of this Element is to guide the reader on the application of robust and easily applicable management strategies whilst dealing with the most challenging aspects of their professional workload.

The authors have categorised various subgroups of emergency neurosurgical workload, devised a comprehensive management algorithm, included case scenaria related to the most challenging emergency situations, and highlighted easily overlooked clinical information. In summary, this Element will provide robust and easily applicable management strategies whilst dealing with the most challenging aspects of the emergency neurosurgical workload.

Keywords: emergency neurosurgery, triage, treatment algorithm, web-based referral systems, on call prioritization

ISBNs: 9781009486026 (HB), 9781009440639 (PB), 9781009440615 (OC)
ISSNs: 2755-0656 (online), 2755-0648 (print)

Contents

Theme

Neurosurgical triage is often the first step in the management of acute neurosurgical patients. A good knowledge base, therefore, of the conditions, timing of triage, and understanding difficulties and priorities is of great value to the duty neurosurgical registrar. Identifying the conditions in need of immediate/ urgent attention, transfer and treatment in timely manner whilst filtering out those which are less urgent or even do not need to come through the acute service all together, minimises the pressures on the limited resources of a regional tertiary centre.

In this Element, after a brief introduction of the UK model triage system, we will elaborate on the cases that require urgent neurosurgical transfer and the timing of transfer, provide an algorithm of a triage system and a decision-making tree, and highlight difficulties and obstacles, including triaging in the post-pandemic era. Additional considerations for the polytrauma patient, the concept of treat and transfer, and finally, the technological development in referring systems and the picture archiving and communication system (PACS) will be separately addressed.

1 Introduction

There is significant variability in the management of emergency conditions across the globe; a good health system model nevertheless offers specialised services. A specialised tertiary centre is a manifestation of increased quality of care, resulting in reduction of morbidity and mortality (1). The NHS model provides tertiary services with a number of specialities commonly bundled together in a strategically located trauma centre serving a number of a regional hospital networks. A neurosurgical unit within the NHS is part of this tertiary system model offering emergency and elective services.

Emergency neurosurgery accounts for 60 per cent of the total workload. The volume and quality of referrals have changed significantly over the last few years (2). The number of referrals has been steadily increasing over the years with an obvious incline in the median age among the referrals age group (3). Better lifestyle choices, patients' education, adapting preventive and screening measures, survival of many diseases including cancer and better prehospital response and care are contributing factors.

2 The Spectrum of Urgent Neurosurgical Conditions

The spectrum of conditions often encountered by the duty acute neurosurgical registrar can be divided into several ways:

2.1 Spinal versus Cranial

This is of practical importance since some centres adopt a separate rota system for the above. Some units have a separate point of contact as well to deal with the volume.

2.2 Adult versus Paediatric

Paediatric units within the United Kingdom are often separate. A particular consideration applies to sixteen-year-old patients. A sound knowledge of the policies specific to the unit is essential to avoid delay in delivering care. However, if the condition is immediately life-threatening, presenting to the ED of the adult centre, it should be treated promptly without any delay regardless of the age. A safe transfer can be subsequently arranged.

2.3 The Relative Frequency in the Referral Database

Traumatic brain injury (TBI) is the most common condition referred to acute neurosurgical services. This is followed by cauda equina syndrome (CES), intracranial space occupying lesions (SOL), and degenerative spine disease. The aforementioned conditions represent 50 per cent of the total volume of referrals. Table 1 demonstrates the cranial and spinal neurosurgical conditions in order of their frequency.

2.4 Based on the Level of Urgency

The conditions highlighted in Table 1 could fall into more than one category. Figure 1 and Section 3.3.1 cover these in detail, but briefly, we need to decide:

Table 1 The cranial and spinal neurosurgical conditions in order of their frequency.

Cranial	Spinal
TBI	CES
Cranial SOL	Degenerative spine
SAH	Spinal trauma
CSDH	Spinal tumours/MSCC
Stroke/ICH	Spinal infection
Hydrocephalus/shunt	Spinal haematomas
Cranial infection	Spinal vascular anomaly
Pituitary	

- Does the patient need to be taken to theatre straightaway? For example, raised intracranial pressure (ICP) such as in severe TBI, stroke, intracranial haemorrhage (ICH), obstructive hydrocephalus, subarachnoid haemorrhage (SAH), and extradural haematoma (EDH).
- If not, does the patient need to come to neurosurgical unit for urgent assessment +/–surgery? For example, moderate TBI, ICH, low grade SAH, infections, spinal fractures, metastatic spinal cord compression (MSCC).
- If not, does the patient need to come to neurosurgery for observation, investigations, and further management? (e.g., moderate/minor TBI, stable fractures, tumours without significant neurology).

3 Principles of Management

3.1 Prehospitalisation

Neurosurgeons rarely get involved in prehospital management; nevertheless, a brief knowledge of this world may help to understand why patients from the same car accidents, for example, ended up in different hospitals! The field crew need to establish a destination after assessing the patient and ensuring the ABCs. This invariably depends on decision-making algorithms, protocols (4). Furthermore, there are a number of point-based systems such as the CRAMS scale; the acronym 'CRAMS' represents the five components measured: Circulation, Respiration, Abdomen, Motor, and Speech. CRAMS is used to help in deciding whether a patient needs to be in the regional trauma centre (5). Prehospital teams currently employ major trauma triage tools to identify patients who may have suffered severe injuries. These tools are based on physiological criteria, injuries identified at scene, and mechanism of injury. Triage-positive patients who are within forty-five-minute transfer time of a major trauma centre are taken directly there, bypassing all hospitals en route unless there is an immediate life-threatening condition such as unrelieved airway obstruction (6). Altering the major trauma triage system in the United Kingdom in 2012 was associated with significant improvements in both the care process and outcomes of patients after severe injury (7).

3.2 The Emergency Department

There are six potential scenarios of interaction as discussed in the subsequent sections.

3.2.1 Life-Threatening Condition Needing Emergency Surgery

The field crew would have contacted the emergency department regarding the condition and the expected time of arrival (ETA). The emergency department will activate a trauma call to the trauma team including anaesthetists with either immediate effect or based on ETA. The patient now is reassessed with primary survey, further stabilisation ABCs, IV lines, intubation and ventilation when needed. CT scan is often needed. The emergency clinician at this point would have contracted the neurosurgical team via the direct bleep (preferability for the life-threatening conditions) or the online referral system if neurosurgeons are not on the ED premises. The presence of neurosurgeon in the ED depends on local trust policies based on the workflow model. It is important to emphasise not to delay transfer if emergency surgery is needed.

3.2.2 Limb-Threatening Condition Needing Emergency/Urgent Surgery

The scenario here may be similar as in major trauma or different such as in isolated spinal trauma, CES, or spinal haematoma. The difference compared to 3.2.1 is that the patient may be (but not always) awake to be part of the dialogue and make decision for themselves. Spinal MRI is needed.

3.2.3 Life-Threatening Condition with Poor Prognosis

The workup is similar to the first scenario; however, based on various factors the general consensus of the decision-making MDT, the patient is not suitable or would not benefit from surgery. Palliation pathway or devastating brain injury (DBI) pathway will be activated (8).

3.2.4 Admission under Different Team/Joint Care without a Neurological Life or Limb-Threatening Pathology

A common example here is a polytrauma patient with skeletal injuries, rib fractures with or without pneumo/haemothorax, and/or with abdominal injuries. The brain and spinal CT demonstrate minor neurological findings such as a small contusion, or a traumatic SAH, or some minor compression fractures. The referring team contacts us to establish a neurosurgical plan (e.g., spinal precautions, ICP monitor, further investigation, delayed surgery).

3.2.5 Referral for Outpatient Management Arrangement

A common scenario is a patient attending the ED for urgent MRI scan which, in turn, does not reveal CES or cord compression, but instead only a small disc irritating a nerve root. Another example is a patient scanned for an unrelated reason and a small vascular lesion or meningioma is found incidentally. An outpatient follow-up or referral to the appropriate MDT is facilitated. *The importance of establishing from the history that the lesion is truly asymptomatic cannot be overemphasised.* In addition, in some units, neurosurgery accepts patients requiring admission for back pain management.

3.2.6 Referral Seeking Advice/Opinion Only

A common scenario here is a patient known to have a previous neurosurgical pathology or surgery and is in the ED for a suspected PE. The ED team or the medical team ask our opinion if it's suitable to anti coagulate.

3.3 Receiving the Referral

Time is of essence once we receive the referral. There is a local policy in place for time of response to the bleep or the online referral. Depending on the level of urgency, the referring team may escalate it to the consultant on call. In response we may either seek further information or if the information is sufficient, we can provide a management strategy.

The instructions should be clear, explained well with justification, and should be based on evidence where and when possible. *We should not underestimate the fact that the referring team will have to convey them to the patient and/or their families.* Therefore, it is useful to provide them with as much information as possible to familiarise them with our strategy. The plan should be discussed and approved by the on-call consultant if it is time-critical or will be discussed later if it isn't.

In case the patient needs to go to theatre, the following applies.

3.3.1 Actioning the Local Transfer Triage

If the patient is in a different unit, the speed of transfer can be communicated using codes making sure the receiver understands those codes as well. This is particularly useful when communicating with ward managers and bed managers. Figure 1 provides an example of transfer triage model.

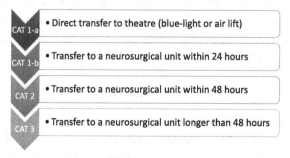

Figure 1 Transfer order triage system model.

3.3.2 Booking Emergency Theatre

Early communication with emergency theatre anaesthetist and staff is very important. The theatre team would like to know the category of the booking; theatre triage is different to transfer triage (cat 1 within one hour, cat 2a within six hours, cat 2b within twenty-four hours, and cat 3 longer than twenty-four hours), the patient details, the proposed procedure, duration of procedure, predicted blood loss, and equipment needed. If emergency theatre is in use, then, can the operation wait, or do we need to open another theatre? If the case is happening in working hours and there is no capacity in theatre, the theatre coordinator will ask if there is an option of disrupting an elective neurosurgical list to accommodate this procedure.

3.3.3 Directing Transfer to Emergency Theatre versus Unit Transfer

Whenever we are transferring directly to the emergency theatre, it is very important to inform the theatre team prior to placing the transfer order, ensuring necessary capacity in theatre. For unit transfers, the unit nurse in charge and/or the bed manager ought to be informed prior to ordering the transfer.

3.3.4 Establishing Order for Polytrauma Patients

Polytrauma patients need special considerations. Discussions between different teams or with the trauma coordinator who may fill this role, establishing priorities and orchestrating the order of the management strategy, are an additional requirement. Figure 2 provides an example of a triage decision-making algorithm.

4 Difficulties and Obstacles

4.1 Availability of Beds and Beds Management

Beds are rarely readily available. Discussing with the ward manager or a bed manager is very useful to establish where the next available bed is, so you can instruct the referring team appropriately. *Never initiate a transfer without knowing the exact destination of the patient.* A patient in the corridor for hours without a designated nurse is not safe! The case scenario discussed in Section 5.3.1 provides a solution to the most challenging dilemma.

4.2 Treat and Transfer

This option is pertinent when there is no chance of a bed in the ICU or neurosurgical wards becoming available. Typically a patient with an acute EDH requiring immediate surgery is operated, and thereafter discussed with adjacent neurosurgical

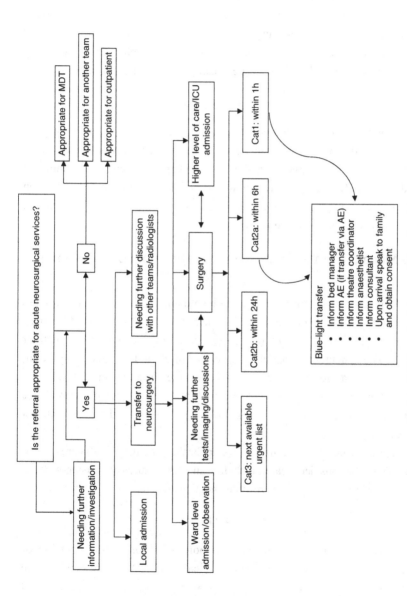

Figure 2 Triage decision-making algorithm.

units for transfer to their ICU for ICP management. Another similar scenario is outlined in Section 5.2.1. The accepting team would require a careful handover of care before and after surgery, including transfer of images.

Occasionally you have to transfer a patient from your local ED to another neurosurgical unit even if they don't require emergency time-critical surgery. In this case, the receiving neurosurgical team may have certain requirements prior to the transfer, such as ICP monitor insertion or a prophylactic EVD. Early discussion with the other neurosurgical team, therefore, is very important.

4.3 Post-Covid Era

The Covid-19 pandemic brought new, unprecedented challenges. We experienced major disruption to patients' care, including elective lists and bed availability. Contingency plans, emergency managerial mandates, temporary guidelines, and protocols were introduced (9) and remain currently in action (10). Familiarising, therefore, yourself with the most up-to-date information in this rapidly changing climate is imperative.

5 Management Scenarios and Variations of Some Common Conditions

Triaging acute neurological cases can be a daunting task. We shall discuss some common management scenarios, including variations that add to their complexity. They represent real cases the authors came across in their career. The management pathways provided might not be the only solution; however, it was felt to be the best at the time. In addition, they may be applicable to some units but not others. Moreover, the scientific evidence and guidelines may evolve or change over time leading to different treatment strategies.

There are a number of general rules applicable to emergency neurosurgery. They should be considered carefully before and during surgical decision-making, and are covered later under the recommendations section.

5.1 TBI

The severity of a TBI is the most important factor on the decision of transferring the patient to the neurosurgical centre. A severe or moderate TBI should be transferred to the neurosurgical centre for neurological observations (neuro obs). A minor and (sometimes moderate) TBI can be observed locally with a clear advice to rescan and rerefer immediately if the consciousness level drops. A life-threatening TBI may be considered for direct theatre transfer taking into account other factors, such as physiological age, comorbidities, anticoagulation and bleeding tendencies, other injuries, current or pre-intubation Glasgow Coma Scale (GCS), and pupillary reaction.

Whilst using the clinical picture remains the corner stone for decision-making along with the radiological picture as an adjuvant aid, some units are developing and adopting point-based systems (11). These systems harness the power of modern computation with genuine promise. Longer-term evaluation, nevertheless, is required before they are adapted into mainstream use.

5.1.1 A Case Scenario

A sixty-two-year-old male patient had an eight feet fall off a ladder on his head. His GCS prior to intubation was E2V3M5. Pupils size 3 equal and reactive. The CT scan reveals a large right acute subdural haematoma, diffuse underlying intracerebral contusions with mass effect, and midline shift. The patient is on clopidogrel for previous TIAs. The haematologist recommended two units of platelets, one at induction and the other one intra operatively, but the lab doesn't store platelets on site. They will arrive from a different hospital which may take a minimum of one hour despite urgent transfer. The patient's pupils are becoming unequal; the right side now is size 5 and non-reactive. How would you proceed?

Solution: Action emergency transfer of platelets and to go ahead with surgery prior to the arrival of platelets. Give tranexamic acid one gram over ten minutes and another one gram infusion over eight hours as per CRASH-3 trial (12). The priority here is that once decompression is accomplished, the intracranial pressure will improve. It is important not to close the wound before ensuring adequate haemostasis. Therefore, you can apply a swab on the wound cavity while you wait for the platelets to arrive.

5.2 Obstructive Hydrocephalus

Obstructive hydrocephalus complicates infections, tumours, and intracerebral bleeds, and requires emergency insertion of an external ventricular drain (EVD). The underlying cause may or may not necessitate simultaneous surgical attention. Insertion of an EVD is one of the most common neurosurgical procedures. However, based on the underlying condition, there are other different surgical solutions to resolve obstructive hydrocephalus; removing a space occupying lesion or an intracerebral bleed in the posterior fossa can restore CSF flow. Some surgeons in other certain conditions elect to place a primary shunt instead of EVD. It is also not uncommon to perform two procedures such as EVD insertion and removal of posterior fossa haematoma.

5.2.1 A Case Scenario

A sixty-five-year-old female patient presented with the sudden onset of sharp pain at the back of her head, nausea, vomiting, and visual disturbance. She quickly became confused and then non-responsive. When she arrived at the ED, she was E1V2M4 with both pupil size 4 and reacting to light. A CT revealed hydrocephalus secondary to a cerebellar infarct. You contacted the ICU consultant and there is no ICU bed available. How would you proceed?

Solution: Treat and transfer. Book the patient for an emergency EVD and decompressive craniectomy. Once the patient's ICP is controlled and is safe, keep in recovery while a regional neuro ICU bed is secured. Make sure you provide a detailed transfer letter.

5.3 Subarachnoid Haemorrhage

SAH is a very common and life-threatening condition that requires urgent transfer to neurosurgical unit. It presents with a variety of symptoms depending on the World Federation of Neurological Surgeons (WFNS) grade. It is very important to establish the WFNS grade after resuscitation and correction of reversible factors such as obstructive hydrocephalus for better prognostication (13). Your duty is to ensure that the patient is safe and stable while waiting for the definitive treatment of the aneurysm, including maintenance of euvolemia, stable mean arterial pressure (MAP), and commencement of nimodipine as per SAH management guidelines; this is one of the few level-A neurosurgical treatment options (14). The surgical management of SAH has changed significantly over the past two decades with the advances in endovascular technologies. Neurosurgeons, nevertheless, have to be prepared to surgically intervene in emergency cases such as hydrocephalus, evacuation of a haematoma with or without clipping, or when interventional neuroradiology is not available or suitable.

5.3.1 A Case Scenario

You have just accepted a thirty-five-year-old female patient with severe headache. Her GCS is 15 with no neurological deficit and pupils are equal and reactive to light. She needs admission for observation for early hydrocephalus secondary to a colloid cyst. The patient may need bilateral EVDs overnight if her GCS starts dropping. The bed manager advised you that she will occupy the last bed in the neurosurgical unit. As you put the phone down with the bed manager, there is a new referral from a regional hospital within your catchment area related to a forty-three-year-old female patient with

WFNS grade 1 SAH. Her CT angiogram shows a large right MCA aneurysm. You contacted the other regional neurosurgical units and there is no bed available in their unit. How would you proceed?

Solution: You urgently transfer the patient from the regional ED to your ED. She will be under the care of neurosurgery in the ED with a comprehensive management plan similar to what would have been received in the ward including neurological observations, fluid balance, bed rest, nimodipine, and analgesia. She will be transferred to a neurosurgical bed when one becomes available or to the ICU for MAP management after her aneurysm treatment.

5.4 Extradural Haematoma

EDH is often a result of a head injury and a skull fracture, almost always acute and very often large and expanding causing mass effect resulting in raised ICP and acutely dropping GCS. It frequently requires immediate surgical treatment although, occasionally a lesion can be observed closely in a neurosurgical unit if the patient is stable with normal GCS and no neurological deficit. Osmotherapy can be useful to gain time while transferring the patient to the preparing theatre. Operating on an EDH in a timely manner is one of the most rewarding conditions for a young neurosurgeon with speedy and excellent results.

5.4.1 A Case Scenario

It is 2:25 a.m. on a Saturday night. You have just informed the theatre staff and anaesthetist that you are booking a CAT1 emergency left craniotomy and evacuation of EDH. The anaesthetic registrar is asking whether it can wait, as they have a patient on table that will take another two hours to finish. You explained that your patient's GCS just dropped from 14 to 11 in the ED, and he has a very large left EDH with significant mass effect and midline shift, and therefore it should not wait. The anaesthetic registrar agrees to open a second theatre and he is calling his consultant. While your patient is being transferred to theatre, your junior doctor calls you to review the patient who was admitted earlier with a colloid cyst who just dropped her GCS from 15 to 12 (E3V4M5). A repeat scan shows worsening of hydrocephalus. She will need emergency bilateral EVDs. How would you proceed?

Solution: You call your consultant to come immediately to operate on one of the cases and you ask the anaesthetist to open a third theatre by calling the second on-call anaesthetist.

6 Technological Developments in Emergency Neurosurgery Triage

6.1 The Utilisation of Web-Based Referral Systems

The use of a secure web-based online referral system has improved communication with other hospitals; referrals are easier, more streamlined, and structured. We can access the system from any suitable location, including the theatre or a secure mobile device. A clear advantage of web-based systems is the provision of rapid access to the wealth of data to draw conclusions on the various parameters. This, in return, helps the health systems to redistribute resources more appropriately (15). Moreover, it has improved the medico-legal aspects through the inbuilt information locking protocols and timing logs. There are, however, a number of downfalls to the online referrals, such as

- The ease of access to a neurosurgical advice which may not be appropriate for acute neurosurgical services.
- The quality of information can be suboptimal or incomplete. This is less likely with telephone referrals as we would have interrogated any pertinent information directly. We can circumvent, nevertheless, this problem by sending follow-up question(s) or seeking clarification(s).
- Technical problems such as system reboot, system failure, or security breaches can compromise patients' safety. Backup plans need to be readily available in these scenaria. The IT team alerts us, invariably, regarding downtimes of planned maintenance or upgrades. Accordingly, it is our duty to convey this information to the referring centres to convert to telephone referrals for the time-critical conditions.

Since the majority of these systems are recent developments, often running as independent businesses with a license agreement with your trust/department, it is useful to familiarise yourself with the system, and have a good communication channel with the system developers and your local IT team. A representative from your department should have regular trouble shooting and quality improvement meetings with the developers. A notebook to record any problem or development idea will be very useful, too. As in many cases, there is an evolutionary curve to the system in order to adapt to your local settings and needs. This topic will be covered more extensively in this series separately (Grundy, Joannides and Ray, *Sources, Modes and Triage of Emergency Referrals to Neurosurgery*, Elements in Emergency Neurosurgery, Cambridge University Press, forthcoming).

6.2 The Interconnected

A PACS is a computerised means of replacing the roles of conventional radiological film: images are acquired, stored, transmitted, and displayed digitally (16). Coupled with progressively developing computational algorithms, it facilitates better understanding of anatomical and pathological conditions. The interconnected PACS enables us to view scans from a very wide range of hospitals (in Scotland for example, the national PACS stores images performed in the entirety of the institutions within the country). It is prone to failure, as almost anything technologically driven, and thus, always be prepared for an alternative option when PACS is down.

7 Recommendations

- Familiarise yourself with local/regional/national guidelines and protocols. If there is no good local induction system in place, consider discussions with other senior colleagues. Never underestimate the local experience of senior staff.
- Do not hesitate to pick the phone and speak to the referring team if you feel the need to do so either due poor-quality online referral or a time-critical situation.
- Ask for help EARLY; Asking for help or advice from your senior colleagues is a useful thing to do and never be too worried about doing so. Always be proactive and do not leave things till last minute or when it is too late.
- The on-call consultant needs to be involved early in decision-making and management. Although majority of non-urgent cases can wait till handover; the few urgent ones should be discussed individually and promptly. After all, it is a consultant-led service!
- Never take a patient to theatre without informing the supervising consultant and documenting his/her plan.
- A multidisciplinary approach is of paramount importance to an emergency neurosurgical decision-making. In addition to discussing with the neurosurgical consultant, it is important to discuss with the ICU team, interventional neuroradiologists (when applicable), and the on-call anaesthetist.
- Whenever possible, try to speak to the patient's family to discuss the condition, the treatment plan, prognosis, and expectations. This is a useful opportunity to understand more about the patient's background as in many cases the ED team did not have the chance to go into the details of the history. Last but not least, you have to ask the patient's personal wishes if they have expressed them to the family members and respect them in the decision-making.

- Careful check of the patient's blood parameters is the responsibility of the surgeon.
- The majority of older patients and some of the younger ones are on some type of *blood thinners*; it is your duty to actively extract this information and advice accordingly. The advice ranges from withholding antiplatelets for a certain period of time to activating reversal. It is not uncommon to seek help from the on-call haematologist specially with the increasing use of non-vitamin K antagonist oral anticoagulants (NOACs).
- The use of osmotherapy will buy us time for transfer or theatre arrangement or repeating scan. But never rely on a 'Good ICP' after osmotherapy. Consider ICP waveform and ICP trend for early decision-making (17).
- Timing of the day plays a role in the surgical planning. It is reasonable to consider a damage control procedure out of hours understanding that the patient may need definitive procedure during 'social' hours. This approach allows better planning, skill mix, and facilities at your disposal during the 'social' hours.

When referred a patient with an 'asymptomatic' lesion, always scrutinise the clinical history: is the lesion truly *asymptomatic*?

References

1. Sahni NR, Dalton M, Cutler DM, Birkmeyer JD, Chandra A. Surgeon specialization and operative mortality in United States: Retrospective analysis. *British Medical Journal*. 2016;354:i3571.

2. Mukerji N, Paluzzi A, Crossman J, Mitchell P, Nissen J. Emergency neurosurgical referrals in the North East of England – trends over four years 2008–2011. *British Journal of Neurosurgery*. 2013;27(3):334–9.

3. Spencer RJ, Amer S, St George EJ. A retrospective analysis of emergency referrals and admissions to a regional neurosurgical centre 2016–2018. *British Journal of Neurosurgery*. 2021;35(4):438–43.

4. Follin A, Jacqmin S, Chhor V, et al. Tree-based algorithm for prehospital triage of polytrauma patients. *Injury*. 2016;47(7):1555–61.

5. Gormican SP. CRAMS scale: Field triage of trauma victims. *Annals of Emergency Medicine*. 1982;11(3):132–5.

6. McCullough AL, Haycock JC, Forward DP, Moran CG. II. Major trauma networks in England. *British Journal of Anaesthesia*. 2014;113(2):202–6.

7. Moran CG, Lecky F, Bouamra O, et al. Changing the ystem – major trauma patients and tTheir outcomes in the NHS (England) 2008–17. *EClinicalMedicine*. 2018;2–3:13–21.

8. Harvey D, Butler J, Groves J, et al. Management of perceived devastating brain injury after hospital admission: A consensus statement from stakeholder professional organizations. *British Journal of Anaesthesia*. 2018; 120(1):138–45.

9. Ashkan K, Jung J, Velicu AM, et al. Neurosurgery and coronavirus: Impact and challenges—lessons learnt from the first wave of a global pandemic. *Acta Neurochirurgica*. 2021;163(2):317–29.

10. Bajunaid K, Sabbagh AJ, Ajlan A, et al. Consensus statement of the Saudi Association of Neurological Surgery (SANS) on triage of neurosurgery pPatients during COVID-19 pandemic in Saudi Arabia. *Neurosciences Journal*. 2020;25(2):148.

11. Gillespie CSN, McLeavy CM, Islim AI, Prescott S, McMahon CJ. Rationalising neurosurgical head injury referrals: The development and implementation of the Liverpool Head Injury Tomography Score (Liverpool HITS) for mild traumatic brain injury. *medRxiv*. 2019:19004499.

12. CRASH-3 trial collaborators. Effects of tranexamic acid on death, disability, vascular occlusive events and other morbidities in patients with acute traumatic brain injury (CRASH-3): A randomised, placebo-controlled trial.

Lancet. 2019;394(10210):1713–23. www.thelancet.com/journals/lancet/article/PIIS0140-6736(19)32233-0/fulltext#%20.

13. Giraldo EA, Mandrekar JN, Rubin MN, et al. Timing of clinical grade assessment and poor outcome in patients with aneurysmal subarachnoid hemorrhage: Clinical article. <u>Journal of Neurosurgery.</u> 2012;117(1):15–9.

14. Pickard JD, Murray GD, Illingworth R, et al. Effect of oral nimodipine on cerebral infarction and outcome after subarachnoid haemorrhage: British aneurysm nimodipine trial. *British Medical Journal.* 1989;298(6674): 636–42.

15. Kennion O, Jayakumar N, Kamal MA, et al. Use of an online referral service for acute neurosurgical referrals: An institutional experience. *World Neurosurgery.* 2022;165: e438-e445.

16. Strickland NH. PACS (picture archiving and communication systems): Filmless radiology. *Archives of Disease in Childhood.* 2000;83(1):82.

17. Meyfroidt G, Bouzat P, Casaer MP, et al. Management of moderate to severe traumatic brain injury: An update for the intensivist. *Intensive Care Medicine.* 2022;48(6):649–66.

Cambridge Elements ≡

Emergency Neurosurgery

Nihal Gurusinghe

Lancashire Teaching Hospital NHS Trust

Professor Nihal Gurusinghe is a Consultant Neurosurgeon at the Lancashire Teaching Hospitals NHS Trust. He is on the Executive Council of the Society of British Neurological Surgeons as the Lead for NICE (National Institute for Health and Care Excellence) guidelines relating to neurosurgical practice. He is also an examiner for the UK and International FRCS examinations in Neurosurgery.

Peter Hutchinson

University of Cambridge, Society of British Neurological Surgeons and Royal College of Surgeons of England

Peter Hutchinson BSc MBBS FFSEM FRCS(SN) PhD FMedSci is Professor of Neurosurgery and Head of the Division of Academic Neurosurgery at the University of Cambridge, and Honorary Consultant Neurosurgeon at Addenbrooke's Hospital. He is Director of Clinical Research at the Royal College of Surgeons of England and Meetings Secretary of the Society of British Neurological Surgeons.

Ioannis Fouyas

Royal College of Surgeons of Edinburgh

Ioannis Fouyas is a Consultant Neurosurgeon in Edinburgh. His clinical interests focus on the treatment of complex cerebrovascular and skull base pathologies. His academic endeavours concentrate in the field of cerebrovascular pathophysiology. His passion is technical surgical training, fulfilled in collaboration with the Royal College of Surgeons of Edinburgh. Finally, he pursues Undergraduate Neuroscience teaching, with a particular focus on functional Neuroanatomy.

Naomi Slator

North Bristol NHS Trust

Naomi Slator FRCS (SN) is a Consultant Spinal Neurosurgeon based at North Bristol NHS Trust. She has a specialist interest in Complex Spine alongside Cranial and Spinal Trauma. She completed her neurosurgical training in Birmingham and a six-month Fellowship in CSF and Trauma (2019). She then went on to complete her Spinal Fellowship in Leeds (2020) before moving to the southwest to take up her consultant post.

Ian Kamaly-Asl

Royal Manchester Children's Hospital

Ian Kamaly-Asl is a full time paediatric neurosurgeon and Honorary Chair at Royal Manchester Children's Hospital. He trained in North Western Deanery with fellowships at Boston Children's Hospital and Sick Kids in Toronto. Ian is a member of council of The Royal College of Surgeons of England and The SBNS where he is lead for mentoring and tackling oppressive behaviours.

Peter Whitfield

University Hospitals Plymouth NHS Trust

Professor Peter Whitfield is a Consultant Neurosurgeon at the South West Neurosurgical Centre, University Hospitals Plymouth NHS Trust. His clinical interests include vascular neurosurgery, neuro oncology and trauma. He has held many roles in postgraduate neurosurgical education and is President of the Society of British Neurological Surgeons. Peter has published widely, and is passionate about education, training and the promotion of clinical research.

About the Series

Elements in Emergency Neurosurgery is intended for trainees and practitioners in Neurosurgery and Emergency Medicine as well as allied specialties all over the world. Authored by international experts, this series provides core knowledge, common clinical pathways and recommendations on the management of acute conditions of the brain and spine.

Cambridge Elements ⁼

Emergency Neurosurgery

Elements in the Series

The Challenges of On-Call Neurosurgery
Abteen Mostofi, Marco Lee and Nihal Gurusinghe

Mild Traumatic Brain Injury Including Concussion
Thomas D. Parker and Colette Griffin

*Models for Delivering High Quality Emergency Neurosurgery in High Income
Countries*
Matthew A. Boissaud-Cooke, Marike Broekman, Jeroen van Dijck, Marco Lee and
Paul Grundy

Acute Spontaneous Posterior Fossa Haemorrhage
Lauren Harris and Patrick Grover

Clinical Priority for Common Emergency and Urgent Conditions in Neurosurgery
Taha Lilo and Ioannis Fouyas

A full series listing is available at: www.cambridge.org/EEMN

Printed in the United States
by Baker & Taylor Publisher Services